Grappling with Grief
and the Pathway to Peace

Jamie Henderson-Warren

ISBN: 979-8-218-30535-2
Published by Aalani Renee Necole/ The Creative Catalyst, LLC

DEDICATION

To my Son:

Calvin Ellis Henderson

March 16, 2015 – April 26, 2015

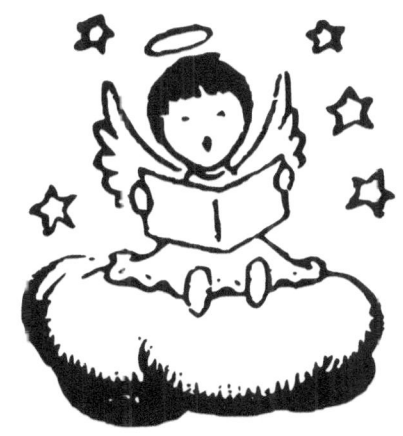

CONTENTS

ACKNOWLEDGMENTS

•

I want to first and foremost thank God for never leaving my side even when I was angriest and pushed him away. Even when I cursed him and abandoned him, he never gave up on me. He brought my heart and soul back to him and helped it heal. He gave me grace and helped me grow with love.

•

I want to thank my Earth side children, Maddison, Owen, and Colton for always being the light of my life. Their love drives me to be the best Mom for them. Everything I do in life is to provide them with the best and all the love I can possibly give.

•

I want to thank my family for staying by my side in my gloomiest days and loving me. For being there when I needed them and even when I felt I didn't and tried to push them away. They have always been there for me, even when I couldn't see it. For always being family.

•

I want to thank my wife Erica for always pushing me to my

best potential. For loving me in my darkness and struggles

and always seeing the light in my soul.

For never giving up on me and always encouraging me.

Always being by my side and walking through life together.

Encouraging me to write this and pursue my dreams. For truly

being my biggest supporter.

•

I want to thank my ex-husband Joshua for everything he did for me

in the depths of the darkest and hardest times of my life. For

putting his grieving on the back burner to take care of me and our

family. I know it wasn't easy, but he put mine first and I will

forever be thankful for that. For giving me four beautiful children.

Thank you from the bottom of my heart.

GRIEF

What do you do when you're living your worst fear? When you feel as though the world has come crashing down around you? When you lose someone you love? Or you lose your career? When you experience loss. When something/someone you cherished or loved is no longer with you.

You have to face what is in front of you head-on. There is no other choice. As hard as it may seem at the moment, remember, this too shall pass.

Everyone's timeline of grieving is different, and that's okay! Some are just coming into it, some are immersed in it, some are coming out, and some are on their path to healing. We all find ourselves in different stages. Whatever stage you are in, as long as you keep pushing, there is hope. The path can be uneasy, but the peace will be worth it. You must want it, you must fight for it, you must fight for YOURSELF!

There are five stages to grief, which we will go through in this book, and how to work through them in a healthy way to find your way on a healing path. I will also be sharing with you my personal experience and my journey through grief. Though our situations may not be the same, we both have experienced grief. You are not alone. Grief is its own to process and work through. When you experience grief, it consumes you. It becomes bigger than you in more ways than you can imagine.

Although we all experience grief in our own time and in different ways, one thing is true…you feel lost. You feel empty and scared. You feel numb. Even if it's for a moment, months, or years, you sit wondering how life will be after a loss. How will anything be the same? How will I be okay? How you handle life after the loss of someone (or something big) is up to you, and on YOUR timeline. A piece of your heart has been taken, but remember it still beats. Although that part of your heart where your loved one is gone, it can come back stronger with time and healthy healing habits.

Whatever stage of grief you are experiencing, this book will provide empathy and reassurance that you are not alone. We are going to explore and go into depth about each stage of grief, my journey through grief, and strategies that may help you on your journey. Ways to help you find your "new normal". Even when you feel low, and like you won't make it through, I am here to tell you that you can, and you will. You must want it though. Simply just doing things to occupy your mind is not healing, that's escaping reality. Its avoidance. The grief will still surface, sometimes when you least expect it. It could be a song, a smell, or even a sound that triggers feelings of grief.

The psyche goes to a dark place and grief overtakes you, even if you are in the best of head spaces, or in the happiest of moods at that time. Unless you allow yourself to work through the stages of grief to truly heal, those triggers will send you into a spiral. That spiral could feel like it's setting you back…and that's okay. As long as you remember to keep moving forward each day in your path to peace and healing, you will prevail. You will learn to recognize and become in tune with your grief, and what triggers it to surface. You will become more aware of what takes your mind to those dark places. However, it takes time and work to find a healing focus to develop and manage ways to cope when it surfaces.

When you experience the loss of a loved one, and in my case my baby boy, you spend so much time looking for answers.

Searching, pleading, grappling for answers. Answers that you will likely never find. Let me ask this question though. If God could give you the answer as to why you had to experience loss, would it help? Would it change anything? Would you grieve any less or any different? These are the questions I started asking myself at the beginning of my journey. Instead of constantly asking and blaming God as to why he took my son, my beautiful baby boy, I now ask, "What were you trying to teach me", and "Did I need to go through all that pain and anguish to become who I am today"? That's not to say those were my thoughts in the beginning and midst of my grief. It was a long road to get to those questions.

The space in my heart that my son occupied might be gone emotionally, but I work every day for him and myself to slowly fill that void. I know that hole will never be as full as it was with him by my side, but it is now filled with less pain and sorrow. I can now say with confidence that I am in a restful state of healing. A stage where I feel, I can continue to grow and thrive.

I'm going to tell you about my loss, the one that sent me into that dark space of consumable grief. Let's start by saying that I lost my child, and I felt I lost a part of myself too. A piece of my

4

soul was taken. What I didn't understand at the time was that the feeling of emptiness was natural, although terrifying. When I suffered the loss of my child, a child I fought so hard to protect. I lost myself. Before this I considered myself to be a strong person, but I felt weak. I realized I would never be the same after this. My mind went to dark places I never thought existed. The morning I left the hospital after they declared him deceased, the world felt different... Although the Phoenix sun was shining as bright as it did every day, I saw only darkness around me. My world felt different. The once-busy noises of the emergency room were now silent. The faces of those around me were blurred due to my tear-filled eyes.

I was about to walk through a hell I never imagined. A hell that would break me down further than I ever thought. A hell that would send my mind and spirit spiraling. This was the beginning of my journey with grief. One that I had never experienced before. It was the beginning of some of the darkest days of my life.

MY STORY

When I found out I was pregnant with my second child, I was ecstatic! I already had one (a girl, Maddison) and now was being blessed with another. Unfortunately, after a few doctors' appointments, that joy turned to fear. I found out I had complete placenta previa, meaning my entire cervix was blocked, and that we would have a long, hard pregnancy ahead.

I was considered a high-risk pregnancy, meaning an early C-section, and lots of bed rest to ensure the safety of myself and my baby. I prayed every day to keep him safe. "Please, Lord let him and myself be safe", "God, please don't let me go into labor early!" I would tirelessly pray every day that my son would make it to a safe delivery. That I would get to see my beautiful baby that I diligently fought to protect. I prayed that the endless days of bed rest, numerous ultrasounds, and doctors' visits would result in a healthy baby!

Then the big day came, he was here! He was born a month early and a big boy at 7lbs 1 oz. Just as I heard his first cry, a tear of relief rolled down my eyes and I thought, "Finally we had made it out of all the craziness". When I asked the nurses to bring him closer and to hold him, I heard and saw them scrambling in nervousness. I saw the look of fear on my then-husband Josh's face. This surely was not the reaction I was hoping for or planned on. I felt so vulnerable and helpless, strapped down to that surgical bed, cut open, and couldn't get to my baby to comfort his struggling cries. I wanted to rip my arms out of the restraints and rush to him. Before I knew it, they were rushing him to the NICU.

The nightmare didn't end there. While in recovery, my mind was trying to grasp that I had just given birth, but my baby was not snuggled against my chest. I was still groggy from the medication, so everything seemed hazy. I couldn't understand how we didn't have that crucial first hour of bonding. Something that made me feel so close to my daughter when I had her. That first hour is when a mother is supposed to snuggle and comfort her child on her chest. They call it the "Golden Hour". I didn't get that.

While resting in my recovery room, a few hours later, I witnessed a team of paramedics, doctors, and nurses holding a

NICU isolation cube with Calvin in it strapped to a gurney. Their demeanor and urgency filled the room with tension. I could feel my heart in my throat. They informed me that my son was in acute Respiratory Distress, and the hospital I was at was not equipped to treat him and he needed to be transported to a higher level of care facility, forty-five minutes away. Shock, terror, and adrenaline kicked in and I began to try and gather my things nervously while grasping the situation going on around me. Still hooked up to monitors and IVs, I went into mama bear fight mode to try to get to my baby. A nurse came over to me to try and calm me down and informed me that he would be going, and I would not. Wait what? She informed me that I had to stay at that hospital to recover, while they transported my baby away from me.

A baby I hadn't even gotten to touch yet. To smell or kiss yet. A baby I fought so hard during pregnancy to keep safe, was just cut from my belly and taken away to another facility. It felt surreal. It felt like I was in a nightmare. It was an excruciating nine days of him being in NICU. I didn't get to hold him until day five. I didn't even get skin-to-skin contact until day six. Almost a whole week had passed that my baby didn't get the comfort of his mother's touch. I knew that if I could just hold him against my skin, he would feel my heart and get better. It really is true when they say that a mother's touch is a healing one. Once I was able to hold him and start skin-to-skin contact, his O2 sats started to improve. He slowly needed less sedation and oxygen push. He was starting to heal. I could feel it in my soul too. We were finally starting to physically connect, and I could feel my baby boy.

Now the hardest part was leaving the NICU every day without him and not knowing when he would get to come home with me, I still felt a sense of defeat. Seeing him hooked up to tubes and struggling to breathe broke my heart. It felt like a distant static noise every time the doctors or nurses tried to talk to me. I just wanted to take my baby home! However, I will forever be thankful for those NICU nurses. They are a special group of individuals to be able to do what they do.

Finally, after nine long days, the day came to take him home! I felt a sense of relief. The days of waiting and countless trips to the NICU to see him were finally over. Tireless nights of pumping to help nourish and strengthen him could turn to exclusively breastfeeding at home. The day was here! I couldn't wait to walk out of that hospital for the last time with him by my side and to never look back!

We finally got to bring our baby home and start a life; I thought hospitals and fear were behind us. All the new baby joys to cherish and experience are now a reality. My daughter, who was almost three at the time, was over the moon to have her new baby brother home to love on. She was so excited to meet, hold, and kiss him. She truly felt like a big sister. It felt like everything was finally starting to fall into place in my life. My family was healthy, happy, and together at home. It was everything I prayed and hoped for. Looking forward, I could never have imagined what was in store for my life and the impact it would have on my family and me.

THE DAY MY LIFE CHANGED

The morning of April 26th, 2015, was when my world stopped and my walk with Grief began. The day/night prior was a busy day, however. We went to my parent's home where my Brother-in-law, who was a photographer, took Calvin's baby pictures. He was so little and curdled up in a red basket with his blue baby blanket that was so soft. My daughter, who was almost three at the time, took photos with him. The Phoenix sun was shining bright and the pictures of the two of them turned out beautiful. It's almost like God knew ahead of time, what those photos would mean to me, so he made the weather perfect just for us! After taking pictures, we went home because we were having some friends over for a game night. That night, I was so exhausted from the day, I had fallen asleep propped up in the bed. My friend that came over for game night slept with us too. I can remember that for some reason that night, my allergies were bugging me. Not thinking twice about it, I laid him next to me, just like I did any other night. Given that he was away from me at birth, and along with it being easier to nurse him, we usually co-slept. With no worry in mind, I kissed my baby goodnight and I fell asleep.

When I woke up the next morning, something was different. I was woken up on my own instead of by my baby cries of hunger. My breasts were aching because it was past the time of his feeding. I went to reach for Calvin so that I could feed him. When I picked him up his face and lips were blue, he wasn't breathing, and I was in shock. An image that is still burned into my brain. All I could do was scream. Panic, terror, and adrenaline hit me like a ton of bricks. I jumped out of bed screaming, "He's not breathing, my baby's not breathing", over and over. I ran out into the living room where Josh and our other friends were all sleeping and continued to scream, "He's not breathing"! Josh took him from me and started CPR right away. One of our friends called 911 as I laid there in shock not knowing what else to do. I was on the ground in the doorway of the bedroom floor feeling so helpless and terrified. I prayed that God would magically heal my baby in the moment and place air back into his lungs, NOW. For a moment, I felt like I was back in the delivery room, and they were taking my baby away from me once again. The same emotions came flooding back into my body.

When a rush of paramedics and firefighters flooded my living room, they took over and started to work on Calvin. I watched as they started hooking him up to all sorts of machines while trying to resuscitate him. They moved so fast that it seemed as if I had blinked, and Calvin was being loaded into the ambulance. To this day, I appreciate their diligence and sense of urgency in their attempt to save my baby boy.

Josh rode in the ambulance with him and I was left to ride in the back of a cop car. It was the worst feeling ever. I felt like a criminal and didn't understand why. At one point we pulled up to a red light and the ambulance raced over the hill and on through to the hospital, but the cop car stayed at the light. I remember yelling, "Please go, get me to my baby!! Why won't you go!?" Eventually, the ambulance drove over the hill, and I could no longer see the lights. Deep down I knew that I would never see my baby again.

While stopped at the light waiting for it to change, I could feel myself almost hyperventilating. My mind was running laps around itself and there was nothing I could do to fix it. I was thinking about how I only had him for six and a half weeks, how I

13

fought so hard through my pregnancy to keep him, and what

tragedy I had woken up to this morning. Immediately, I realized

that life could change in the blink of an eye.

DENIAL

There were still so many initial questions racing through my brain. Did he roll over and couldn't roll back? Did my friend move wrong and make the blanket roll him into me? Why didn't he cry to wake me when it was time to nurse? Why didn't I just take a nap or not have people over, so I wasn't so tired? Was this my fault? I could go on for days with ways I was racking my brain trying to rationalize what was happening. The realization that death is real and is a part of life, is terrifying! The permanency of death can bring up feelings of regret. When we lose people close to us, we immediately start to wonder, was I nice enough, did I say I love you enough, or why didn't I call them when I had the instinct to do so. I was walking right into denial.

I didn't know much about grief before that morning, at least not to the extent of what I was experiencing. They say the loss of a child is unlike any pain ever felt or experienced, and it's true. It's unlike anything that I can put into words. Parents aren't supposed to outlive their children. Parents aren't supposed to bury their children, plain and simple. Yet here I was in that exact predicament. I literally felt like I was living in hell on earth. I was not mentally, emotionally, or spiritually prepared for this journey I was about to embark on. I was not prepared to endure the grief journey, and to be honest, at this time, I didn't care to learn about it either. I was terrified and angry. I was in uncharted waters and didn't know how to move forward.

So, let's get into denial. This is the first stage of grief, which I have to admit was one of the hardest. Fear, guilt, and anxiety are but a few of the common emotions we feel in this stage. When we experience loss, we struggle to believe that our loved one is really gone. I remember thinking day in and day out, this isn't happening. I will wake up and this will all be one big, realistic nightmare. The thought that your loved one is gone stirs up a deep, heavy feeling in the pit of your stomach. I often tried to redirect my thoughts to avoid facing the reality that my baby was no longer a part of the physical. I would think to myself, he was just here with me and now he's not.

During the stage of denial, we don't feel that our psyches

have had enough time to process the reality of what we are experiencing, and in all honesty, it hasn't.

When we returned home from the hospital that morning, I went into his room and just sat next to his crib that we had finally put together the day before. As I sat in a room surrounded with his things. I kept telling myself that he was just at the hospital. I wanted myself to believe he was back in the NICU, and I would be able to go and bring him back home soon. Even with everyone hugging me and crying, I still struggled to believe that he was gone forever. Looking back, I realize that I was still in shock. It could not be real that I would never get to watch him grow up. I would never get to kiss his squishy cheeks again. It couldn't be real that my little squish was gone.

Denial almost gives us a sense of relief. If we allow ourselves to believe that what we are experiencing is not real, it hurts a little less, at least in the moment. During the denial stage. I can remember feeling frustrated because I didn't see other people feeling what I felt. Was I wrong to think that others should be hurting as bad as I was?

Denial shows up in different forms and for everyone, it may look a little different. I thought that when I went to the funeral home to prepare for his funeral, I would face the reality of his passing. I was planning a funeral for my baby, surely that would be a sign that he was gone, right? Wrong. Even sitting there picking out his urn and flowers, I still refused to believe that this was real. I kept thinking I would wake up from this nightmare and my life would go back to how it was supposed to be. At one point the funeral director called me to set up my final viewing and told me to bring a beanie for him because of the incision around his head from the autopsy. This wasn't enough for me. I still thought it was a nightmare and damn it, I was ready to wake up from it.

So, I know you're wondering, when did it finally hit you? When did it become a reality for you? It didn't feel real to me until we entered the chapel and I saw his lifeless body lying on the altar so peacefully. Suddenly, everything that I was in denial about hit me like a ton of bricks. I dropped to the floor and just started screaming, crying, and yelling. My then-husband and Calvin's father, had to pick me up and physically walk me to the altar.

When I gathered the strength to place my eyes on him, he looked so serene, yet so still. I placed my lips on his cold cheek, and it sealed the deal for me. There was no more life left in his little body. My baby was truly gone…this was real.

The following days consisted of me putting on a fake smile. People would come and go, offer their "thoughts and prayers", and go on with their lives. As the days grew longer, I grew number, literally. The next week I had my OBGYN six week follow up, in which I had to attend without Calvin. After informing her of the tragedy, she saw it fit to prescribe me medication to help with my high levels of anxiety and depression. This appointment was so hard for me to even attend because I knew I would be showing up without my baby. They even had to cover all the baby announcements on the walls of the room because it was physically too hard for me to look at. My baby should have been up on that wall, but instead I was there alone.

So, here I was. Unable to continue living in denial and having to face the reality of child loss. I couldn't escape it any longer. My baby was gone and there was absolutely nothing I could do to bring him back. For you, it may be the loss of a spouse and sleeping in an empty bed or losing a Grandparent and no longer receiving birthday calls. It could be losing a pet and no longer having them at the door to greet you with a wagging tail when you get home from a long day of work. Trying to call your loved one, and they don't answer. Going to their house and it's empty. Or ultimately attending their funeral and seeing the casket. Reality hits us all differently.

When experiencing denial, give yourself GRACE. You're not going to be okay today or tomorrow. You may not be okay a month or a year from now, but what I can tell you is that each day that you push forward, it will hurt a little less. Feel your emotions. Try your best to refrain from pushing them away. Trust me, I tried this, and it only made things harder for me. During this time, I truly wish that someone would have told me that it's okay to not be okay. When reality hits you and you are at a loss for what to do next, the first step is to put one foot in front of the other and move forward little by little. Your journey of grief will be ran at your own pace. This process is not a sprint, it is truly a marathon. Spend as long as you need to in denial, but you can't stay there forever. It's your decision to be a prisoner of grief or you can decide to walk your imperfect journey not allowing grief to lead the way. You are the only person who has the power to determine your grief and how long you experience it. Remember, every person has different coping strategies and what works for one person may not be what helps you. Find what works for you! For me, it was journaling. Journaling gave me an outlet to express my thoughts, feelings, and emotions safely, even if it didn't make sense at the time. It was something I could reflect on at a later date to see where I was and how far I had come. It was a way to express myself even when I couldn't get literal words out. It may even help you too. Now that we have covered denial, let's move on to the next stage of grief, anger.

ANGER

Anger can take over your mind, but only if you let it. It can have a negative impact on your relationships, health, mind, body, and soul. We all feel and experience anger differently as it can show up in a variety of forms. Some may ask, what is anger, truly. Anger can be defined as a strong feeling of displeasure, hostility, or annoyance. When we feel anger, we have a plethora of physiological responses. Some may experience an excess amount of sweat. Others may experience a red face and destructive behaviors. It's beneficial to know and understand how your body responds to anger so that you can recognize when you are experiencing this emotion. This level of self-awareness also gives you the ability to cope appropriately.

When I lost Calvin and anger kicked in, I found myself angry at God, angry at the world, and most of all, angry at myself. I was looking high and low to find someone else to blame, but in reality, there was no one. I spent many days and nights trying to rationalize why my baby was taken from me. Not only that, but the way he was taken from me. Later, I learned that I was seeking control. To seek control is when we try to grasp an understanding of a specific situation. We didn't have control of how we lost someone or the circumstances, and we don't have control over our emotions following the loss. Truthfully, we will never understand why and that makes us even more angry!

It is important to remember that we can't control everything. It's easy to feel weak when we can't control things, however.

Last chapter I mentioned that others don't really feel the pain we feel when we lose someone significant. Some may feel it in different ways. Although this can also contribute to our anger, it's important to remember that most of the time, no one will ever know how you feel about certain situations. When in your presence, others may pose the question "Why are you so angry with me, I'm just trying to help". While this may be true, they may just not quite understand how to help. This is where we really need to keep a healthy and reliable line of communication open with the people that we love. It's normal to want to push people closest to you away in times such as this, however, we never truly want the people we love to feel as though we are pushing them away. This only fuels anger on both sides.

During my experience with the anger stage of grief, I pushed everyone away. Looking at people just made me angry because I knew I would never get to look at Calvin in the physical again. When others wanted to help, I took it as they were trying to fix me, not be there for me. Several people told me that I needed to seek professional help so that I could have someone to talk to. Couldn't they see that I didn't want to talk to anyone? Wasn't it obvious that I was angry? I was nearly drowning, and I was not ready to come up for air. All I wanted was for everyone to leave me alone. Deep down inside I wanted to tell them to shut up and go away. I wanted them to realize that they would never know how I was feeling and because of that, they wouldn't be able to help. Even in a crowd, I felt alone and ultimately, I wanted to be alone.

My deepest anger was with God. How can you be the almighty who has the power to bring the dead back to life, but you allowed my baby to die right next to me? Why make this experience a part of my life if your plan is not to harm me? Now I'm confused, I'm hurt, I'm angry, and I just want answers. I did everything right. I fought for him tooth and nail like a mother is supposed to do for her child. He didn't deserve this and neither did I. Why didn't he just take me? I was racking my brain every second of every day trying to find out what I did wrong to deserve this torment. In my mind, God was my enemy, not my savior. I was furious. I felt abandoned, alone, and hurt and he allowed this. There was no light left in my soul, only anger and hatred. It was overwhelming.

At this point, anger began pouring into my marriage. My husband and I started to blame each other for this tragedy. Our grief was projecting onto one another, and we struggled to express love and comfort, the thing we needed most from one another. Sometimes we would find each other angry at the other simply because we felt that more grief should be displayed. We started to believe that the other didn't care as much because certain actions or behaviors were not aligned with what we thought grief should look like. During this time, there was a lot of yelling and fighting.

We would isolate and avoid each other more and more. My husband suggested that we begin marriage counseling ASAP. In my mind, I was wondering why he was ready to move on from this when I was still in such mourning. I felt like he wanted to forget about Calvin and just move on with life and I wasn't ready to endure that. I wanted more time to mourn. Him suggesting counseling made me even more angry. I agreed, but not wholeheartedly. I wasn't mentally ready; I carried Calvin in my womb, how could he ever understand the connection we had?

It took a while, but I finally realized that I was being selfish. He was hurting too. I mean, Calvin was just as much of his son as he was mine, how could he not be hurting? I forgot to pay attention to his emotions. I was so consumed in my own anger and sadness that I didn't recognize the strength that he had been displaying for my daughter and for myself since everything happened. In this moment, I realized that I had let anger have the final say. Anger was controlling me, my thoughts, and my behavior.

While I can admit that I lived here for a while, I eventually found my way to the other side. I realized that anger had a huge impact on my relationship. I could have done a better job at communicating with him. I believe had I gotten outside of myself to communicate, I would have been a better support for him and my daughter. This was not the catalyst that drove my divorce, but I truly believe that it played a factor.

So, in this moment, I want you to ask yourself, "What can I control?" Two things that I realized I had complete control over were my actions and my reactions. I couldn't control what I was going through, and I couldn't control how people "supported" me, but I could control how I reacted and received it all. When I came to this realization, I was able to start working on controlling my anger. Granted, I didn't wake up one day and all my anger had disappeared. It took time. A long time!

Day by day I began working on letting go of control. I would notice my negative thought patterns more and more. As I noticed them, I tried to redirect them. When I felt myself falling back into anger, I thought about at least one thing I could be grateful for. This was not easy at first, but it got easier as time went on. This takes a certain level of consciousness and consistency. Take it from me, falling back into old thought patterns is much easier than changing them. Anger and peace do not coincide. It's one or the other and only you have the ability to make the choice on which one to focus on.

Anger is natural and it has the power to interrupt your path to peace. Healing is impossible when you choose to operate from a place of anger. It's important to find local grief support groups to help you appropriately cope with grief. When my family encouraged me to talk to someone, I resented them. I never got the courage to genuinely talk to someone but looking back I wish I had at the time. I can say that my experience influenced me to counsel others and support them on their journey, because eventually, I learned the importance of having support. Talking to someone takes a great level of courage and commitment but is so worth it.

Remember, people want to help you! They may not have had the exact experience that you had but they can act as an outlet. People are willing to listen to you without judgement. Don't allow yourself to get frustrated when you slip back into the anger stage.

It is normal. This can be extremely hard around anniversaries or holidays. Feel your emotions, address them, and move forward in the best way you know how. Your emotions are valid. Lean on your support system as they are a part of your solid foundation and will help keep you accountable. Not only that, but they will also provide a great line of support for you as you strive for healthy healing on your path to peace.

BARGAINING

This stage is where the "what ifs" and "if only I did…" start to consume your brain. Then you drive yourself crazy trying to play out different scenarios which ultimately only circle you back to anger. Angry because you can ultimately not control the realistic outcome. You might find yourself racking your brain with these questions to the point that you would rather give up something or even yourself to have that person back. If you are religious or believe in a higher power, this is when you start to try and make a deal with God.

You will encounter yourself ruminating over what could have gone differently or what you could have done to avoid the loss. You sometimes start to play out different scenarios in your mind that involve the loss of the person you are grieving for and different outcomes. Your mind just wanders. This simply is a way for you to hold on to hope that the person may not actually be gone, but deep down, we know that's not true. You try to convince your psyche that if you can bargain and give up something in return, then maybe your loss won't be real.

This is a stage that most might not find themselves dwelling long in but is one that should be recognized. You start to focus on thoughts within the mind and begin devising ways in which things could have been or gone differently. Essentially you are in turmoil with your psyche. This can be a very confusing stage because deep down you know these "deals" or "bargains" you try to make with a higher power are unrealistic, but you also long for them to somehow be true. That somehow if you "become a better person" or "a better Christian" and "if I just convince God I will do better", then all of a sudden, you and your loved one will be reunited, and it will all just have been a dream.

This is the stage that can create a lot of daydreams, where we get lost within our own mind. We may be finding ourselves replaying memories of that person, or loss and trying to come up with various circumstances in which the end result isn't what the truth is. However, the truth is still there. Under all the daydreams, mindless thoughts, and unheard prayers and conversations. The truth is still that the loss occurred, and we must endure the path ahead. It is not to say that this stage is not beneficial or detrimental. It's that this stage is unrealistic. This is the stage we go through where our memories of that person and perhaps our last encounters are replayed over and over. Sometimes it may feel like torture to have these memories on repeat, but it's your mind's way of imprinting that person into your forever psyche. To help you later remember the good times and even the bad. It's a way for you not to forget that loss, but to embrace it.

For me, this stage is not one that I spent a lot of time in. I am a realist and even in the midst of my grief knew there was nothing to do to bring my son back. It's not to say I didn't spend time in this stage, because I did. I would find myself spending countless hours replaying that night and morning. Thinking of things, I could have done differently. "What if I took a nap", "What if we didn't have friends over", and "If only I had put him in the bouncer". These are thoughts and questions I would drive myself crazy with. I tried to re-play every last-minute detail to see if there was something that I missed or could have done differently that would allow me to still have my baby.

I would scream and cry at God and beg him to take me instead and bring my son back. I would plead for another chance to just hold him or kiss him. All things that I knew were not humanly possible, but my mind wanted to believe. I wanted to hope that somehow a miracle would happen.

This occurred the most while we were at the hospital that morning, and a team of doctors, nurses, and EMTs were all in one little room trying to bring him back to me. It was a small amount of time, but felt like forever while they worked on him. I cried and screamed and bargained with God. "Please, just let him live and start his heart". Then, to all their best efforts as they did everything they could, I finally heard the doctor say, "I have to call it…Time of death 0637". I saw the defeat in everyone's face and that's when I lost it and physically broke down.

My pleading and screams were not heard, my desperate prayers went unanswered, and the nightmare became my reality. As they all walked out of the room, the doctor came up to us and said "Sorry…", but everything became so fuzzy. It felt like I was living outside my body watching all of this happen. We went in to give him a last kiss and it was as if I felt myself watching this outside of my body because I don't believe my soul and psyche could handle the realization. I called my parents from the hospital and told them, but all I could get out was "Calvin is dead." The screams of my mother and hearing my father in the background still pierce my soul. Their first grandson was no longer here. They had just held him the night prior, and then the next morning they were hearing of every parent's worst nightmare and unsure of how to navigate forward for us and for themselves. Once we left the hospital, I realized my barging at the moment was unsuccessful. This was when the torturous replay of "what ifs" began to flood my brain as I sunk into the next stage, depression.

DEPRESSION

The word depression is used so often today that sometimes it can be hard to understand what depression really is. It can be easy to mistake sadness for depression and depression for sadness. According to the National Institute of Mental Health, depression is a mood disorder that displays severe symptoms affecting how one thinks, feels, and handles their activities of daily living[1].

Depression is powerful and has the power to drag us down and make us feel like we're suffocating, literally. It's a different type of beast. Depression can be considered one of the longest and hardest stages of grief. When experiencing depression, it's normal to isolate yourself from the world. When consumed with grief, alone time is necessary. We aren't ready to see and face the outside world yet. It gives us the opportunity to process an intense situation. Being depressed after a loss is completely normal and is nothing to be ashamed of or embarrassed about. It is a raw part of the process and something that should be recognized,

---

[1] National Institute of Mental Health

acknowledged, and properly treated. Depression can become detrimental when we sulk here and deter help. This can look different for everyone.

I remember my struggle with depression after losing Calvin. There were days I didn't want to get out of bed to shower or eat. All I wanted to do was lay there and mourn. All I could do was cry. It all felt so heavy and often unbearable. My brain felt like mush. They say your brain is such a powerful thing, but it was at a loss for how to cope with what I was experiencing. My life was in utter disarray and my world was dim. This stage of grief was the longest and hardest stage of my pathway to peace. For me, depression was a mix of numbness, feeling lost, guilt, shame, hatred, failure, and intense sadness. I had no desire to feel better and eventually started to believe that this is who I was, and this is how my life would be from here on out.

From the house that I never returned to again due to the tragedy, I only took Calvin's blue baby blanket that morning. It still had his sweet baby scent on it. It was the only thing I had left of him, and I was not letting it go. When we got to my parents' house, I went straight to their bed and that is where I stayed for days, crying. When I went to the bathroom, you better believe that the blanket came with me. That blanket, for some reason, was the only thing that made me feel a sense of peace. Eventually, my baby's scent wore off the blanket. I knew it would be a sad moment when I realized his scent was no longer lingering but a healthy push to move forward.

I, being the stubborn woman that I am, had convinced myself that I could fix this on my own. As time went on, I tried everything to numb the pain. I wanted this intense pain to go away so I began drinking heavily. It was the only thing that could make me feel better in the moment. It erased my pain temporarily and I found myself not thinking of the tragedy as much. It was my band-aid, my crutch. Drinking was an ongoing struggle for me for quite some time. All I wanted to do was feel better and fill the void I felt inside of me. Drinking was a way to escape my pain, my reality, and people around me. This was an ongoing coping strategy for me however, it almost destroyed me. I didn't know how to ask for help and at this point, didn't think I needed any help. No matter how many of my loved ones told me I needed help, I was so engulfed in myself and my misery that I ignored them all. I had truly convinced myself that everything was okay, and even that I was okay. I was living in a perpetual self-destructive cycle.

One day I had a life-changing decision to make. I was either going to keep drinking and lose everything and everyone I loved, or I was going to ask for help and move forward. I knew that I could no longer do this alone. I realized that there was no possible way for me to continue drinking and work through my emotions with a clear mind. Not to mention, I still had a husband and daughter that I needed to be present for. I was already nonexistent for too long. At one point I remember thinking that I would be better off dead. How could I not stop to think about the daughter that I would be leaving behind without a mother? The pain that I would ultimately just be passing on to her and those around me. Depression had my thoughts as hollow as they ever were. I knew that being sober would be painful because I would have to feel every emotion all over again, but I knew I had to. I would have to process everything with a clear mind and that scared me.

Eventually, I worked up the nerve to ask for help. I realized that my problems and emotions were bigger than myself and if I was going to face them, I needed help to do so. In this moment it dawned on me; I have a little fight left in me. I can still be strong for my daughter and my family all while being present. Most importantly, I can still fight for myself. I wanted to make my son proud. I knew it was not going to be an easy process, but nothing worthy ever is. I began to feel ready. I found a desire within myself that wanted healing and peace.

It was time to focus on my mental health, rebuild myself, and stop succumbing to my grief and depression. Yes, Calvin is gone, but at least I still have memories. Six and a half weeks of memories. I knew that we would be unable to create more memories with him, but at least I could hang on to the ones I had. That didn't mean I wouldn't continue to feel emptiness or sadness. It simply meant that I had to take that reality and move forward. I knew that those cherished memories I had would one day be easier to smile upon. One day I knew I would find joy there!

The reality that that person is gone leaves us empty. It is an emptiness that maybe you have never felt before, or one that you have gone through, and it brings back a flood of uneasy memories. Either way, when we are dealing with a loss, we feel an emptiness in the absence of that person. All the memories that you once had with a person are simply that, memories and so you choose to hold on and cherish them. I know they will be painful to think of at first, but one day when you're further along in your path, they will bring you joy. They will bring a smile back to your face. It will light up your heart with who they were and the love you had.

As mentioned earlier, depression is powerful. Giving depression control leaves us stuck, powerless, and ashamed. It takes over our lives. When depression is in charge, it feels like there is no way out. Something to remember when experiencing depression on your grief journey is that you can, and you will find joy again. Depression is not permeant and there is a way to the other side. Depression is but a bridge on your path to peace. It is up to you to decide how the ramification of depression will affect your life. Most importantly, NEVER be afraid to ask for help! I'm going to say that again because it is very important. NEVER BE AFRAID TO ASK FOR HELP!! You are not alone, and people want to help you. Yes, there's a stigma around mental health and asking for help but let me ask you something. When we break a bone, we are expected to go to the doctor, right? When we are sick, we are expected to visit a professional, right? What's the difference when our brain's feeling sick and overwhelmed? GET HELP! We have convinced ourselves that asking for help is a sign of weakness, but it is the complete opposite. It takes courage, strength, and bravery to ask for help.

Healing and working through this stage cannot and should not be forced. You, and only you know when you are ready to move forward. There is no timeframe for this. Asking for help reflects that you have recognized that your struggles have become bigger than yourself and you need help. Being able to process your grief during the depression stage is much better when you feel heard and supported. When you remember and are reinforced that your feelings are valid. That your sadness is understandable and to have someone to listen and work with you as you heal. How is that weak? I will leave you with that question as we move on to the next stage of grief, working through and accepting.

WORKING THROUGH AND
ACCEPTANCE

Although grief feels impossible to work through at first, we eventually find ourselves at a place where we're ready to accept reality and move forward. This stage is called acceptance. When I think of acceptance, I think of being creative. Here, I found myself exploring different strategies and utilizing appropriate resources that worked best for me. I encourage you to do the same. When we implement or create strategies that work best for us, we seem to commit to them more and for longer periods of time. These strategies can include coping skills, support groups, talking with a therapist, or even journaling. I recommend finding more than one strategy that works for you so that you have more than one tool in your toolbox. For instance, we may not feel like working out or exercising every single day, especially when we are having a rough day. Instead of working out, we may just lay in bed and journal to express our emotions instead. By using more than one strategy, not only are we keeping our toolboxes full, but we also open the door for grace. It's easy to talk down on ourselves or feel guilty when we are doing something that we feel we should be doing or have committed to.

WORKING THROUGH

When working through grief, there will be a multitude of emotions that's felt. Some of these emotions may have been experienced before, but others may be new to you. Working through grief feels like we are rebuilding our lives one day at a time. Each day will bring something new, both good and bad. Some days will be more painful than others. Sometimes it may even seem like no progress has been made. Even when it feels impossible and the pain seems unbearable, there is a piece of strength left inside of you that will allow for you to work through your feelings and emotions. If you've never heard the song "A Little Bit Stronger" by Sara Evans, I highly recommend it. Although it references a breakup, Sara Evans digs into working through the hurt and pain she's experiencing. There are snippets of this song that remind me that no matter what, day by day, I get a little bit stronger.

Have you ever felt like when you put forth effort in certain situations something tends to knock you back? Spiritually, this can be what we refer to as the enemy, or Satan. On the grief journey, triggers can be our enemy. My biggest trigger was, and can sometimes still be, a song. When my son passed, it was around the same time that Paul Walker passed. When I first heard the song "See You Again" by Wiz Khalifa", it deeply resonated with what I was feeling. It triggered such deep and painful emotions for me. For some reason, this song would take over my conscious state. One day I was driving around Phoenix, Arizona, where I lived at the time, and this song was on the radio. I looked around and realized that I was passing the hospital where Calvin was declared deceased. Before I realized it, I was sitting in an unknown parking lot forty-five minutes away from home. I had no recollection of the drive after passing the hospital and hearing that song. I was terrified because I had never experienced anything like this before. Actually, terrified was an understatement. Looking back, I realize that I had experienced a form of disassociation. From this point on, this song triggered me so deeply that I would immediately change the radio if it came on. If I was grocery shopping or in a store and the song came on, I would drop everything I was doing and leave. This song literally had the power to send me down a rabbit hole that I never wanted to go down again. It had a sense of control over me. That song was my plague and I avoided it at all costs.

It was not until I took the initiative to face my fears of feeling deep emotional pain again that I could listen to that song and fully feel the emotions of it. This didn't happen overnight. It took three years to gather the courage to do this. Three years after the passing of Calvin, I was sitting in the parking lot of the Pick' N Save grocery store, loading my groceries I had just bought. Low and behold, I hear this song playing on the radio. Instinctively, I wanted to rush to the front of the car to change the song, but it's like God whispered in my ear and told me listen to it. While listening, I wept. I begged Calvin to forgive me for not protecting him. I apologized to him over and over. I cried as hard as I did when I lost him. I felt every raw emotion I had. It was in that very moment that I relinquished all control to my emotions and to that song.

When the song went off, I prayed. I spent more time talking

to God and Calvin. I started to feel a sense of relief. I hadn't felt relief since it all happened, but in this moment, I felt something that I can hardly put into words. From this point on, that song didn't have as much control over me. To say that I listened to it every time it came on would be a lie. Honestly, to this day, I will sometimes change it when it comes on the radio. The determining factor in whether I listen to it or not is how I'm feeling in the moment it comes on. If I'm not in the right mindset to hear it, I respect that and change it.

You will experience setbacks, especially when working through your emotions. When I experienced emotional setbacks on my journey, I realized that the more I was in tune with my goal to obtain peace, the less the triggers knocked me off track. I found that although I couldn't control what triggered me, I could control my reaction to those triggers. I was eventually prepared to face, or work through, each emotion as they came. It wasn't easy. It took a lot of conscious and intentional effort to get here. Your peace can take as long as you need it too, remember there is no timeline. You will find your way.

ACCEPTANCE

Accepting the loss of a loved one doesn't mean that you're "okay" or that you have forgotten the loss. Acceptance means that recognition of reality has taken place and that moving forward is possible. During this stage, you may feel a little more vulnerable and can accept that you need a support system. The feeling of acceptance isn't necessarily a euphoric one, but I must say it is freeing. When we accept things and choose to work on ourselves, we get closer and closer to peace. Acceptance allows for barriers to be removed and chains to be broken. Accepting the loss of a loved one leaves us with memories, but also the realization that memories can bring us joy. Once I accepted reality, talking about Calvin became easier. It didn't feel as raw, and it started to hurt less. In fact, talking about him now helps me keep his memory alive. The memories I allowed myself to block out now bring me happiness and peace. I have accepted that for his birthdays and holidays, my family can allow for his memory to live on through celebrations and traditions. Acceptance has allowed for me to even discuss with others the emotions I felt throughout this process, hence the writing of this book.

I mentioned in previous chapters that a coping strategy that really helped me was journaling, but I wanted to touch on it a little more here. I found comfort in journaling because it allowed me the opportunity to write down and acknowledge what I was feeling, in a private setting. Some may think of journaling and the traditional "Dear Diary..." comes to mind. I didn't find it to be that way in my experience. Sometimes I would write paragraphs or pages and other times I would write a sentence or two. How much you write or what you write is merely your decision. When I would hear "See You Again", sometimes I could only write as much as, "Today I had a horrible day. I heard his song and I felt so many negative and painful emotions. All I could do was spend hours crying". Sometimes I just wrote, "Today was rough, but I made it and am grateful I didn't feel as sad as yesterday". There were times when emotions or thoughts would cross my mind throughout the day, and I would just jot them down in the notes section of my phone. In today's society, phones seem to be the one thing we don't leave home without. Make it a beneficial object to have in your grieving process.

Journaling also provided me with the opportunity to see my progress on my journey. Some days I just take the time to go back and look at my past journal entries. Doing this gives me a sense of happiness knowing that I've come so far. To see how broken I was in the beginning to how I maneuver now validates for me that God is real. That my feelings and emotions were valid. Some entries are very hard for me to read because I know how I felt and I remember what it was like, however, it's inspirational because I overcame a lot to get where I am today. I clawed, I fought, I screamed, I cried, I pushed people away, but I also grappled my way to the other side of grief.

Now that we have an overview of what working through and acceptance can look like, let's keep in mind that what worked for myself and/or others, may not be what works for you. Time frames of healing will look different for everyone so try your best to stay focused on yourself and avoid comparison. Comparison is the thief of joy and can take you all the way back to the beginning. Instead of comparing, try writing down what you are grateful for daily. Remember, as we grapple with grief, we are exploring and discovering our new normal. You can and you will discover a new meaning of life. This experience, though it sucks, can make you stronger and better equipped to deal with difficult emotions in the future.

Work hard to recognize your triggers. Triggers are dangerous and you may discover on your journey that triggers exist that you never knew existed. Write them down along with ways to cope with these triggers. This is an ongoing process but one worth committing to. We never want to hurt someone we love because they unintentionally triggered us. You have worked so hard to get to this place. Don't let a trigger defeat or control your reactions.

Work hard for yourself. You are worth it. God can do immeasurably more than we can ever think or imagine, BUT we have to meet him halfway. Never give up on yourself and by the grace of God, peace will find you. God will restore you! Give yourself grace on this journey, especially in the working through and acceptance stage. You will start to rebuild your life one day at a time during this tough stage, but soon your days won't be as consumed with tears, pain, and sorrow. A brighter light will start to shine on you.

A piece of my heart and soul were taken from me on that morning and it is something that can never be replaced. With acceptance, it has become a little easier for me. My son will forever be in my heart, but I have accepted that this is where he will stay until God calls me to be with him again. Okay, let's move on to the next chapter, Forgiveness.

FORGIVENESS

Forgiveness is something that I wanted to touch on because although it's not considered to be one of the stages of grief, it is something many of us experience, or will experience, on our journey to peace. According to the dictionary, to forgive means to let go of anger, or resentment, caused by an offense or mistake[2]. Have you ever had to forgive someone who cut you deep? It doesn't happen overnight. I think we can also agree that forgiveness allows healing to come forth a tad bit quicker.

"I forgive, but I won't forget", is such a contradictory statement in my opinion. Holding on to something that uproots anger and resentment within you is not beneficial. When experiencing grief, it is easy to shut everyone out and sulk in our own feelings of guilt, regret, and shame. Our emotions tend to compound until they can no longer be contained, much like we experience in the anger stage of grief. Finding it within ourselves to forgive breaks the chains anchoring us to sadness, depression, and anger. Though grief is natural, forgiveness is not. It requires a

[2] https://www.dictionary.com/browse/forgive

decision, effort, and a certain level of openness in our hearts. Forgiveness takes courage, but from experience, I can tell you that freedom is on the other side and life feels just a little lighter.

Although I had worked through all the stages of grief, I still didn't feel complete. I still felt like I was holding on to so much sadness and pain. At this moment I came to God. It was time to forgive him for what I believed to be him taking my son away from me. When I made a commitment to forgive myself and God, I unlocked a new stage of life. I did not blame him anymore for taking my son, because I knew Calvin was safe in his arms. This realization allowed me to feel sorrow but maneuver my way through it without blame and guilt. Through the darkness, I was able to see a future. I felt hope again. I knew that if God forgave me, I could forgive me. I started to believe that I was worthy of forgiveness.

When working through forgiveness, I realized that I blamed myself more than anything or anyone. I blamed myself for not protecting Calvin. I blamed myself for relying on alcohol to get me through hard times. In the process of forgiving myself, I recognized that I coped the best way I knew how in that moment.

I'm a true believer that if we have the skills to do better, we do.

Since I lacked skills to do better, I felt like a failure. I also realized

that although no one blamed me to my face, others blamed me too.

In heated arguments with my ex-husband, married and divorced,

he blamed me for Calvin's death. He said such hurtful things that I

internalized and allowed them to bring me down further. In these

moments, I would think, how could he blame me? Did he not know

I was already going through hell and blamed myself? Did he not

see me hurting? Instead, he's blaming me for our son's death. If no

one else understood the turmoil I was living in, I thought that he

should. Instead, he was so cruel when he was angry.

Then, I did not stop to think that this was his way of

coping. He was sad and hurting and I did not stop to see that

because I was so consumed in my own grief. Blame can make

someone feel better in the moment but can cause so much damage

to others. I now realize that although it wasn't healthy, he was on

his own journey, and this was his way of working through his

grief. Like any husband would, he spent so much time putting his healing aside to take care of me, that his emotions had been suppressed all along. I will always be grateful for the emotions and pain he put on the back burner to be the leader of the family because I know I was not strong enough at the time to do so. Even though we are no longer together, we walked this path of sorrow alongside one another. I am forever grateful for the strength he showed and for taking care of me despite his own feelings not being validated. We now have three beautiful children together and I will cherish them every day I am alive. It has been a journey for us, but even though we aren't together we are still on a true healing path alongside one another. We know that to be the best parents to our children we had to forgive each other. It took a long time, but now we show each other grace.

Forgive yourself for disrupting caring and positive relationships that were sent to support you. Forgive yourself for not being a good friend, wife, mother, father, brother, sister, etc. Grant yourself the same Grace that God grants you because you are worthy and deserve that. I know you are angry with how things turned out. I was angry at myself for not doing the things I thought

I should be doing to protect Calvin the night he passed. I know you're confused and scared. I was confused and scared when I woke up to my baby not breathing. I'm going to say it again, FORGIVE YOURSELF!

Sometimes it's others that we blame for our grief experience. Work hard to forgive those you negatively associate your grief with. Forgive the doctor who gave the diagnosis, the person who was driving that, the babysitter who wasn't watching your child close enough. Whoever it may be, find it in your heart to forgive them. This may take time, but I promise it will be freeing. Forgiving them is not for their gratification but for your self-resolution.

I say all of this to say, forgiveness gave my life meaning again and I believe it can do the same for you. I didn't know where to begin, but I did it anyway. I chose forgiveness over being a victim and I want to help others do the same. We all deserve a life of peace and happiness no matter our circumstances. I want you to feel the peace that's destined for you. Today, I receive what I believe to be signs from God that my baby is safe and watching over his family. White butterflies remind me of Calvin and God sends them my way often. When seeing them, I feel reassurance and peace. I will forever be a mother to Calvin, and he will forever be a son to me. Knowing this brings me peace, and knowing I will see Calvin again in heaven. I will be able to hold and kiss him and tell him all about his family's life. I will be able to tell him the love we always had for him. I will be able to show him how my experience on earth with and without him strengthened my soul and lead me to peace. That I healed. Take a moment to think about what brings you peace. Write it down and place it somewhere you'll see it every day. Manifest your peace because it is waiting for you on the other side of forgiveness!

A NEW NORMAL

As we approach the ending of this book, I wanted to reflect on a few key points discussed in earlier chapters. In August of 2023, I was driving back from Charlotte, NC after attending a Beyonce concert, which was absolutely amazing by the way. I went to YouTube and searched for a sermon to listen to on the drive and I ran across Sarah Jakes Roberts, the daughter of the amazing Pastor T.D. Jakes. The sermon was titled "Push Through". She asked several questions while preaching but one question stood out to me most: Where is your openness? In what areas of your life do you feel open and how do you fill that opening?

As I reflected, I thought about my experience with losing Calvin. I had to ask myself "How was I filling my openness. Was it a positive filling? Was I using negativity to fill an empty void to satisfy myself and others? What was I doing to avoid the enemy's destruction that I have endured? Am I living in my new normal with a peaceful mind and heart?"

Hopefully these questions of self-reflection will impact you as much as they have impacted me. I encourage you to take time to think about how you are filling the openness of your mind and heart. What we listen to, what we say, and what we fill our time with matters. If it is not serving you at the highest level or not supporting you as you grapple your way to peace, you may need to reevaluate it. This could mean letting go of, or taking a break from, friends and family who are not pouring into you and helping you move forward. As hard as it may be, you need to reflect on that.

When experiencing grief, we are very vulnerable and open. In this place of vulnerability, things like people, media, and social media have the power to influence our decision making, good or bad. Protect yourself and feed yourself with information that will fill your cup. Finding your new normal includes coping with pain, negative thoughts, sadness, anger, depression, and fear or anything that triggers you. It includes questioning whether your decision to forgive someone or something was worth it for you. Finding your new normal is having the conscious awareness to replace negative habits and coping skills with more positive ones.

I encourage you to try things like helping others. You can do things like volunteering or starting a support group to help others through their early stages of grief. You've been there and others are where you once were. Be grateful for where you are because there was a time that you prayed to be here. Others need you so don't be afraid to take a leap of faith and guide others! Pray for and with people. You have experienced God's Grace, and you now know what it looks like to experience it and live it. You can help others recognize grace and accept it on their pathway to peace.

Celebrate the loved one that you lost. This could look like saving a special piece of their clothing and pulling it out from time to time to feel the comfort of them. Watching a show that you all used to watch together or one that makes you smile when you have a thought of them. Work hard to replace the negative experience of losing them with a positive thought or action that brings a smile upon your face. Remember it's okay to tackle the trauma of losing them with the help of a professional.

I celebrate Calvin by being a Mental Health Therapist. I

find joy, fulfillment, and comfort in helping others. When I cross paths with clients who are grappling with grief, I first offer an empathetic ear. Most times, people just need to be heard without judgement. To know that their feelings and emotions are valid. When I find it necessary to share my experience and journey with others, I do. It is not always necessary though. Every day I try to be a reflection of God's Grace and serve others. I believe that I experienced the loss of Calvin for a reason and in remembrance of him, I never want to miss my calling of helping others through their experiences. I never feel the need to rush or force someone to move along in their grief journey because everyone grieves in their own way and every person's timeline is different. This doesn't make anyone's grief less important than another. It simply makes it thier own.

Another way I celebrate Calvin is by releasing balloons every year on his birthday. Out of all the special days in the year, I must say that this is the hardest for me, year after year. Even today, it hurts knowing that I'm celebrating a day for my baby, but without my baby. In the past I would get a cake, but it seemed to hurt more knowing that he wasn't here to blow out the candies and make a wish. Once I realized this was not the way I wanted to feel on his birthday, I implemented a new celebratory act. A balloon release required no cake, no song, no party, and no candles. It was a way for me to celebrate my baby but not give myself enough time to fall back into the early grieving stages. Now for his birthday, I write a heartfelt letter, tie it to the balloon, say a prayer, and send it off to heaven. Not only is this a way for me to keep his memory alive in me, but my children get excited on his birthday because they get to participate in his balloon releasing celebration. Even though Calvin came and left before my youngest two boys, they are aware of who he is. I reassure them that it's okay to talk to him and tell him everything they want him to know, and they do. I also encourage them to ask me anything they want to know about him. Even though it hurts to know they never got to know their big brother, I know that I can keep his memory alive by telling them how beautiful he was. During balloon releases, the kids will say, "Let a balloon go to Heaven for brother". This makes my heart smile.

This celebration can be harder for my little girl as she was alive but young when we lost Calvin. She often speaks of faded memories of him, but she was only three years old when he passed. She briefly remembers how sad mommy and daddy were during this time but can now celebrate his life with a smile. She enjoys writing letters to him and connecting them to her balloon like mommy. Something I learned from this experience is that your children learn from you. They learn to mourn how you mourn and often times will celebrate and smile about things they see you celebrating and smiling about. I knew that isolating and shutting everyone out on Calvin's birthday yearly, would only pass it down to my children so I changed the narrative for them.

Although I experience days that are harder than others, I've learned appropriate ways to cope with those days. My babies see me upset sometimes and when they ask, I'm not afraid to tell them that I've been thinking about Calvin, or that something reminded me of him and made me sad. I want my children to know that it's okay to feel sad. I also remind myself to appropriately model how to handle these feelings, because if you have kids, you know they pick up on everything! My babies will know that their mom is strong! She experienced grief in its darkest form but came out on the other end to be a better person for the people she loves. Calvin is no longer here, but I know he would want me to be the best mom I can be to his siblings. That drives me. He is always in my heart, and I will always have an open space for him there. I have learned to cherish the short six and a half weeks I had with him instead of mourning the loss of him so deeply. More days than not, I feel peace.

Always remember that your pathway to peace is yours and yours alone. Your new normal is one that you can create, good or bad. It will look different for everyone so never compare your path to someone else's. We have acknowledged our loss and accepted it while working through our stages. We have forgiven ourselves and others, the best we know how. Now we must think about what that new normal life looks like. Never quit fighting! Keep going and you'll realize each day you get a little bit stronger. Putting one foot on the ground in the morning is a reflection of your strength. You will always have good days and bad days, and some will be harder than others, but always try to find gratefulness on your journey. Day by day, each morning breath will become fresher and stronger. Acknowledge all steps in your process, whether big or small. Applaud yourself every chance you get because you are enduring the strength to overcome the pain day by day. From me to you, always fight for yourself, trust in God, and never give up. I wish you love, happiness, and a graceful path to peace!

ABOUT THE AUTHOR

Jamie was raised in Phoenix, Arizona but now calls Eastern Tennessee her forever home. She attended Sandra Day O'Conner High School and then went on to Northern Arizona University where she studied Criminal Justice with a minor in Sociology. She has always had a compassionate heart and wanted to help others. She has three beautiful children on earth with her and one in heaven. Madison, Owen and Colton keep her very busy and active. She is currently pursuing her Master's in Clinical Mental Health Counseling and hopes to one day open her own practice. She currently works in behavioral health at an inpatient hospital in which her love and passion for mental health grew. When she is not working, she enjoys spending time with her wife Erica, children and their two dogs, Milo and Lilah, being outdoors, coaching her daughter's basketball and embracing the peace. She hopes to help others who have suffered a lost and remind them they are not alone!

REFERENCES

1. (https://www.nimh.nih.gov/health/topics/depression.com)
2. https://www.dictionary.com/browse/forgive.com

Reflection Questions:

1. When I feel upset, I can contact…

2. I experience sadness most when…

3. My grief journey has taught me…

4. My biggest regret is…

5. If I could say something to you, I would say…

6. What are some ways you have expressed grief in the past? Were these expressions hurtful or helpful?

7. Some activities or healthy coping skills to engage in that help me feel better…

8. Five things I am grateful for….

9. Thoughts of grief that come up often…

10. Ways to celebrate my loved one includes...

NOTES

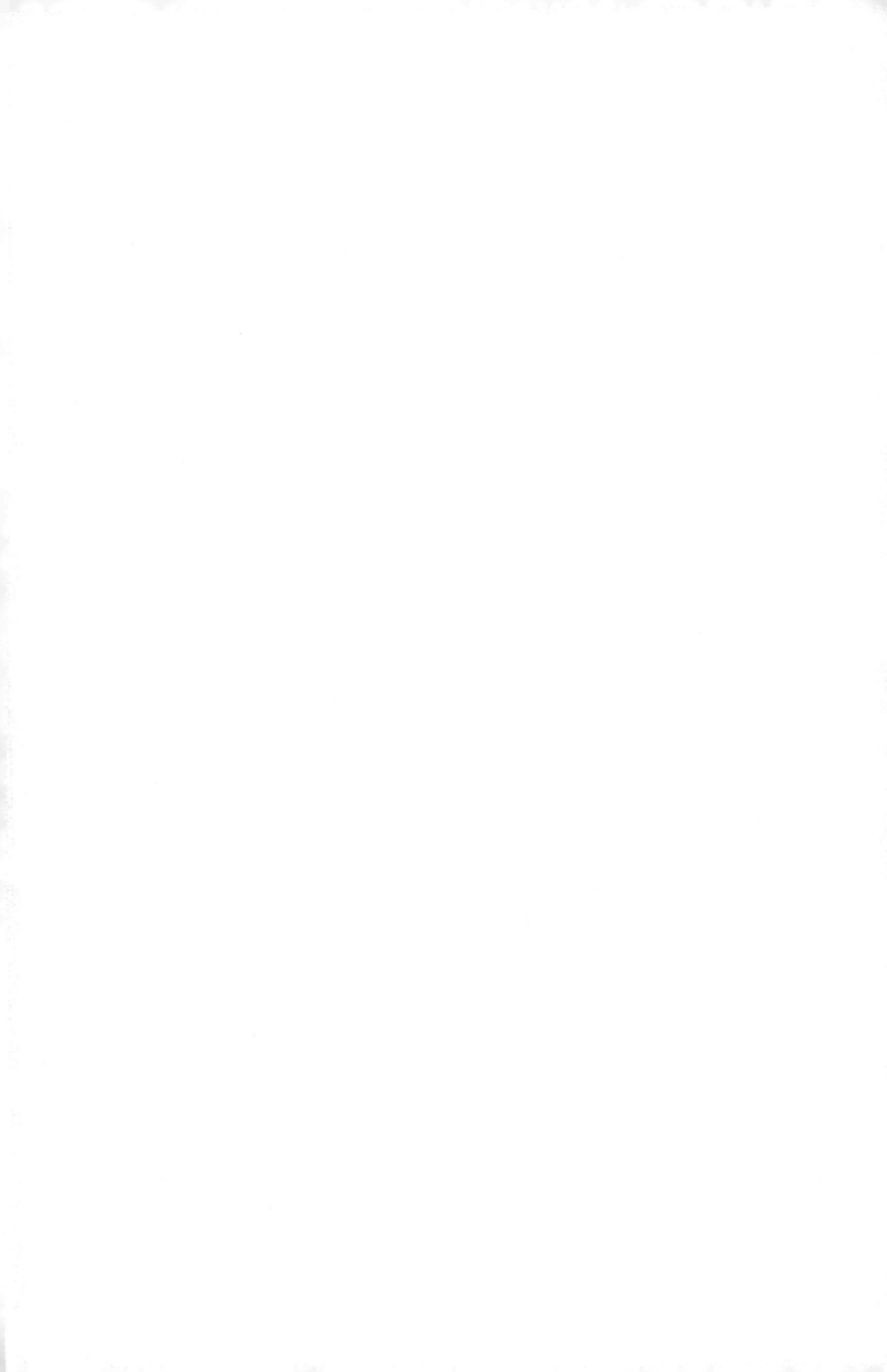